CU00842362

The Better Bath v Fragranced Bath Salts

Written by Lacey Jones

Disclaimer:

The information contained in this book is for general information purposes only.

While we endeavor to keep the information up to date and correct, we make no representations or warranties of any kind, express or implied, about the completeness, accuracy, reliability, suitability or availability with respect to the book or the information, products, services, or related graphics contained in the book for any purpose. Any reliance you place on such information is therefore strictly at your own risk.

None of the information in this this book is meant to be construed as medical advice. It has not been evaluated by the Food and Drug Administration.

Essential oils are powerful compounds. Consult with a medical professional prior to making changes that could impact your health.

Contents

Chapter 1: Introduction to Fragranced Bath Salts

If you're like me, there aren't too many things you enjoy more than a long soak in the tub after a hard day's work. It doesn't matter whether you've just finished working long hours on the job or have spent all day cleaning house and taking care of the kids, you deserve a relaxing bath at the end of the day. That long soak can be made even more luxurious by adding fragranced bath salts to the tub. The water you're soaking in will be conditioned to the benefit of your skin, the salts themselves will help you relax and wind down, and the essential oils used to fragrance the salts will fill the room with great scents while providing a number of benefits to your skin, your body and your state of mind.

Those who purchased volume 1 of my Better Bath series of books learned how to make bath bombs that provide a number of therapeutic benefits. This volume teaches you how to make fragranced bath salts that are simple to make and have many of the same therapeutic properties. Toss a handful or two of bath salts into the tub, and they'll dissolve and disperse their contents into the water. All you have to do after that is settle in for a wonderful bath time experience.

When you make your own bath salts at home, you have ultimate control over what goes into your bath salts, so you can ensure they're made with natural and healthy ingredients, unlike some of the bath salts sold in stores. While there's something to be said about a great-smelling bath, your baths will be even better because they'll smell great and they'll be good for you. What more could you want?

While I'm sure you'll love using the bath salts in this book, don't stop there. People love receiving fragranced bath salts as gifts. They can be made for a lot less than what it costs to buy them in stores, so you'll impress your friends and family members when you start giving containers of bath salts as presents. You can also package them up and sell them at boutiques and you can even sell them online.

Chapter 2: The Main Ingredient

It should come as no surprise that the main ingredient found in bath salts is. Salt is the number one ingredient.

What does surprise people is the vast number of designer salts that can be used to make fragranced bath salts. These salts can run the gamut from inexpensive salts like Epsom salt to very expensive and hard to find designer sea salts. Steer clear of table salts and other salts that have additive like anti-clumping agents and iodine. Table salts aren't a good choice to use to make bath salts.

There are two types of salts that are commonly used to make bath salts. *Sea salts* are obtained by evaporating water from the sea. Most sea salts are named after the sea or ocean from which they're obtained. *Mined salts* are taken from mines dug deep within the earth. Most mined salts come from areas that were once vast seas and have since been covered over with dirt.

There are a wide variety of salts that are sourced from places all over the globe, from the Himalayas to the Pacific Ocean in California. For the most part, the salts used in fragranced bath salts can be used interchangeably. If a recipe calls for Himalayan pink salt, you can probably get away with using a cheaper salt like Epsom salt and still get something that's passable. It's up to you whether you want to invest in the more expensive salts.

The salts that are used to make bath salts can add the following benefits to the bath:

- **Cleanse and detoxify the skin.**
- **Ease muscle cramps.**

- Help alleviate pain and stiffness associated with arthritis.
- Improved circulation.
- Pain relief.
- Relaxation of the nerves and muscles.
- Relieve stiffness in the joints.

Let's take a look at some of the more common salts used to make fragranced bath salts.

Epsom Salt

Epsom salt is named after a "salt" spring located at Epsom in Surrey, England. It's called a salt, but it technically isn't a real salt. It's made up of a blend of magnesium and sulfate that looks similar to salt in its crystallized form.

As far as bath salts go, Epsom salt is by far the most popular salt used in the bath. It's a soaking aid that can be used to help relieve minor aches, pains and general stiffness. It's got calming properties and is a great salt to use when you want to settle in for a nice relaxing soak in the tub. The magnesium and sulfate found in Epsom salt is easily absorbed into the skin, and once inside the body it helps regulate enzymatic activity while reducing inflammation and improving nutrient intake. It also helps the body remove toxins from the system.

The best thing about Epsom salt is it's one of the least expensive bath salts on the market, and it's easy to find. It can be purchased for a buck or two per pound and is sold at pretty much every department store, discount retailer and drug store in existence. Failing that, you can buy it online, but it'll cost you a little bit extra after factoring in shipping costs.

Dead Sea Salt

Dead Sea salt is salt that's taken from the Dead Sea, which is a large sea that's bordered by Israel and Jordan. It differs from salt derived from ocean water in that only around 3% of Dead Sea salt is sodium chloride, while refined table salt is somewhere around 97% sodium chloride.

Commercial Dead Sea salt is obtained from the mud of the Dead Sea and is packed full of minerals and other beneficial compounds. A soak in a tub with Dead Sea salt in it can help stimulate blood circulation and may be an effective therapy for rheumatoid arthritis and osteoarthritis. It's also thought to be an effective home remedy for a number of skin disorders including acne and psoriasis. It helps moisturize the skin and may be instrumental in eliminating rashes and inflammation.

Dead Sea salt works well in fragranced bath salt recipes and won't break the bank. Expect to pay between $3 and $5 per pound for this salt.

Himalayan Salt

Himalayan salt is an ancient salt that's been buried since Prehistoric times. It's taken from mines dug deep into the Himalayan Mountains and comes from large salt beds that were once part of an ancient sea. Over time, the seas disappeared and great mountains formed where the seas once sat. Himalayan salt is made up primarily of sodium chloride, which means it's almost pure salt. There are a handful of other compounds in it, including iron oxide, which is what gives it the pink color it's known for having.

This salt is considered by many to be the gold standard as far as bath salts are concerned. It can be purchased in a variety of grades, ranging from fine powder to extra-coarse crystals. I've found the best salts for bath salts lie somewhere between the extremes, and I prefer medium to small grains. The larger grains can be used to create bath salts that look amazing, but in practice don't dissolve as well as the smaller crystals when tossed into the tub.

The most popular variety of Himalayan salt for bath salts is Himalayan pink salt, which has a light pink hue. It tends to be more expensive than most other salts, but it still isn't going to break the bank. Look for sellers that sell in bulk, and you'll be able to get it for as little as a few bucks per pound if you buy larger amounts. Steer clear of the designer boutiques that package this salt in pretty packages and charge a premium for it.

Designer Sea Salts

There are a ton of other sea salts on the market that can be used to make bath salts. Most of these salts work well, but your mileage may vary.

Some of the designer sea salts out there can get a bit pricey, depending on where they come from and whether or not they're the in thing at the time. To be completely honest with you, I've tried some of the more expensive salts, and they didn't seem to be any different than the previous options.

The only time I use a different salt than the ones we've discussed is when I find one that has an interesting look or color. Sea salts can be found that are naturally-colored blue, pink, grey, red, yellow, black and a number of other colors. Just when I think I've seen it all, I find a different awesome color. Of course you can always just dye one of the white sea salts to make it the color you'd like, but where's the fun in that?

Chapter 3: Borax in Bath Salt Recipes

Spend enough time researching fragranced bath salt recipes and you'll undoubtedly come across recipes that call for borax as part of the recipe. It's added to recipes because it acts as an emulsifier and a buffering agent. It's also a great natural preservative that can extend the shelf life of the products that contain it.

While I don't have a problem with natural borax being used in bath products, many of the online recipes I've seen don't differentiate between natural borax and the commercial-grade borax sold by most stores. Commercial borax sometimes has chemical surfactants and detergents added and is anything but natural.

If you decide to add borax to your bath time routine, only use natural borax that's intended for cosmetic use and keep the amount used to a minimum. Take care when handling the borax. Always wear gloves and avoid inhaling the particles. It can cause irritation if it comes in contact with the skin, your eyes or your mucous membranes. Keep it away from your kids and your pets. When the correct type of borax is used in the proper amount, the end result may be softer water and clean skin. The key is to make sure you're using cosmetic-grade borax and that you're using it in the right amount.

I've avoided using borax in the recipes in this book because it can be a mild skin irritant for some people and I'm not looking to make bath salts that withstand the test of time. It isn't because I'm overly worried about it...I just don't see any need to include it in my recipes. There are some questions as to whether borax can cause problems with fertility and whether it can do harm to unborn children, so those looking to get pregnant or who are already pregnant should avoid it at all costs.

Chapter 4: Adding Fragrance to Bath Salts

Fragrance can be added to bath salts in one of two ways. It can be added in the form of *fragrance oils*, which are synthetic oils that add chemical fragrance to the salts, or it can be added in the form of *essential oils*, which are natural compounds taken from plants that smell like the plants they're taken from.

When fragrance oils are used, they're added for no reason other than to add fragrance to the bath salts. They smell good and there are a ton of different options to choose from, but they don't add anything other than a good smell to the bath salts. The biggest problem with fragrance oils is they're often made from proprietary fragrance blends, and the consumer is left with no clue as to what's inside the oils. You could potentially be using compounds that shouldn't be coming in contact with your skin.

Essential oils, on the other hand, are entirely natural compounds that smell great and carry with them a number of benefits. They aren't without risk, as certain oils can cause problems when they come in contact with the skin and there are oils that shouldn't be used by pregnant women and people with certain health conditions, but there are a number of essential oils that are considered safe for most people to use. I almost always opt to use essential oils in my recipes unless I'm trying to make a bath salt recipe with a fragrance that isn't attainable through use of essential oils.

The best part about essential oils is they add therapeutic benefits to the recipes they're added to. Essential oils can do everything from alter your mood to helping your skin and body function more efficiently. Less is more when it comes to using essential oils to fragrance bath salts. All that's usually needed to fragrance 4 cups of bath salts is 15 to 30 drops of essential oils. Individual oils can be used or you can combine the oils into oil blends that stack a number of benefits into a single blend.

Chapter 5: The Basic Bath Salt Recipe

Here's a quick and easy bath salt recipe to get you started. This recipe doesn't call for any particular essential oil or oil blend. We'll get to those in a bit. Instead, it leaves the essential oils used up to you. It's a great recipe to use when you're experimenting with different oils and oil blends because it's simple and easy to make. All you need is salt and essential oils.

The type of salt used in this recipe is left up to you as well. I recommend starting with Epsom salt or one of the cheaper sea salts until you've found an essential oil or oil blend you like. Once you've got it dialed in, you can start experimenting with the more expensive salts if you'd like.

The Basic Bath Salt Recipe

Ingredients:

4 cups natural bath salt
15 to 30 drops of your favorite essential oil or oil blend

Directions:

1. If you're using an oil blend, combine the oils before adding them to the salt. If you're using a single oil, move on to step 2.
2. Combine the bath salts and the essential oil or oil blend.

3. Stir the essential oils into the salt until the essential oils have completely dispersed into the salts.
4. Spread the salts out and let them dry.
5. Store them in a nonreactive container in a cool, dry place.

Chapter 6: Lavender Bath Salts

It seems like every single book on natural bath products that use essential oils starts off with a recipe that has lavender. At risk of being too cliché, this book is no exception.

Lavender essential oil is one of the most popular essential oils in existence, and it's mild enough to where it can be used by most people. It carries a number of benefits with it, from being good for the skin to being a calming and soothing oil that can be used to help you wind down after a long day. Since lavender essential oil blends well with most other essential oils, this recipe can be used as a jumping off point for experimenting with oil blends. Try blending citrus oils, wood oils or other floral oils into this recipe to see what you can come up with.

The type of salt you use in this recipe is left up to you. I personally prefer Dead Sea salts, but you can just as easily use other natural bath salts and get good results. If you want to dye this recipe, a small amount of natural purple soap coloring will do the trick nicely.

Lavender Bath Salt Recipe

Ingredients:

4 cups natural bath salt
20 drops of lavender essential oil

Directions:

1. Combine the bath salts and the lavender essential oil.
2. Stir the essential oil into the salt until the essential oil has completely dispersed into the salts.
3. Spread the salts out and let them dry.
4. Store them in a nonreactive container in a cool, dry place.

Lavender Sprigs and Salt Recipe

This recipe builds on the previous recipe by adding crumbled dried lavender sprigs. They're there pretty much just for aesthetic purposes, but they also add more fragrance to the recipe.

Ingredients:

4 cups natural bath salt
½ cup dried lavender sprigs, crumbled
20 drops of lavender essential oil

Directions:

1. Combine the bath salts and the lavender essential oil.
2. Crumble the lavender sprigs and stir them into the bath salts.
3. Stir the essential oil into the salt until the essential oil has completely dispersed into the salts.
4. Spread the salts out and let them dry.
5. Store them in a nonreactive container in a cool, dry place.

Relaxation Blend

This recipe adds Bergamot essential oil to lavender oil to create a soothing bath salt blend that will help you unwind. A cup of this in the tub after a long, stressful day will help you forget about your worries and prepare for bed.

Ingredients:

4 cups natural bath salt
10 drops lavender essential oil
5 drops Bergamot essential oil.

Directions:

1. Combine the lavender and Bergamot essential oil.
2. Stir the essential oil blend into the salt until the essential oil has completely dispersed into the salts.
3. Spread the salts out and let them dry.
4. Store them in a nonreactive container in a cool, dry place.

Chapter 7: Tea Tree Oil Bath Salts

Unless you've been living off-the-grid for the last few years, you've probably heard of tea tree oil. While knowledge of tea tree oil used to be limited to aromatherapists and those with knowledge of home remedies, it's managed to make the move into mainstream health and beauty products. While many of the commercial products don't contain enough actual tea tree oil to make a difference, this recipe can be used to add plenty of tea tree oil to your bath time routine.

Tea tree oil comes from the tea tree plant and has a medicinal smell that you probably won't care for at first. I'd heard all sorts of good things about tea tree oil before I smelled it for the first time, and once I finally got a bottle of it, I was shocked that anyone would use a product that smells like that. Luckily, the smell grows on you, and most people learn to love it and the benefits that come with it. Tea tree oil can be used as a home remedy for a number of skin conditions, from acne to fungal and bacterial infections. It's been used as a home rememdy for lice, athlete's foot, MRSA and dandruff. Inhaling steam containing this oil is said to help relieve congestion and may help alleviate the symptoms of the flu and the common cold.

Tea Tree Oil Bath Salt Recipe

Ingredients:

4 cups natural bath salt
15 to 20 drops of tea tree essential oil

Directions:

1. Combine the bath salts and the tea tree essential oil.
2. Stir the essential oil into the salt until the essential oil has completely dispersed into the salts.
3. Spread the salts out and let them dry.
4. Store them in a nonreactive container in a cool, dry place.

Chapter 8: Eucalyptus Bath Salts

If you've ever meandered through a eucalyptus grove and enjoyed the fragrance of the eucalyptus trees, you'll probably love this bath salt recipe. It will fill your bathroom with the fragrance of eucalyptus thanks to the campherous eucalyptus oil contained inside.

Eucalyptus essential oil has a medicinal fragrance that punches right into your sinus cavity. It can be used when you have a cold or a respiratory condition to provide at least some relief. Breathe deeply while you're sitting in the tub and you might find your breathing is less labored. This oil is a stimulating oil that will leave you feeling refreshed and awake.

You might notice that there is less eucalyptus oil added to this recipe than what we've been using when other essential oils are used. Eucalyptus essential oil is considered a warm oil, and it isn't well-tolerated by everyone. Start with a small amount of oil and check to see if you can tolerate it. If so, you might be able to up the amount used, but do so at your own risk.

Use natural soap coloring to color this recipe green for added visual effect if you plan on giving it as a gift or selling it.

Eucalyptus Bath Salt Recipe

Ingredients:

4 cups natural bath salt
10 drops of eucalyptus essential oil

Directions:

1. Combine the bath salts and the eucalyptus essential oil.
2. Stir the essential oil into the salt until the essential oil has completely dispersed into the salts.
3. Spread the salts out and let them dry.
4. Store them in a nonreactive container in a cool, dry place.

Eucalyptus Mint Cold Busting Blend

This recipe takes the previous recipe and ups the cold busting power by adding peppermint essential oil to the mix. Be careful when using these bath salts, as the two oils combined create a potent one-two punch that not everyone can handle. A short soak is usually all that's required to provide relief.

Ingredients:

4 cups natural bath salt
10 drops of eucalyptus essential oil
5 drops of peppermint essential oil

Directions:

1. Combine the eucalyptus and peppermint essential oils.
2. Combine the bath salts and the essential oil blend.
3. Stir the essential oil blend into the salt until the essential oils have completely dispersed into the salts.
4. Spread the salts out and let them dry.
5. Store them in a nonreactive container in a cool, dry place.

Eucalyptus Vanilla Blend

At first glance, this is a combination that doesn't seem like it would meld together, but for some reason, it works great. Adding vanilla completely changes the way the eucalyptus smells by adding an interesting vanilla note that dances in and out of the campherous eucalyptus fragrance.

Ingredients:

4 cups natural bath salt
10 drops of eucalyptus essential oil
½ teaspoon vanilla extract
1 teaspoon Grapeseed oil

Directions:

1. Stir the eucalyptus essential oil, vanilla and the Grapeseed oil together.
2. Combine the bath salts and the essential oil blend.
3. Stir the essential oil blend into the salt until the essential oil has completely dispersed into the salts.
4. Spread the salts out and let them dry.
5. Store them in a nonreactive container in a cool, dry place.

Chapter 9: Herbal Bath Salts

Herbal bath salts take the same herbs and spices that are used in food recipes and adds them to bath salts to create interesting fragrances. You can add the herbs themselves by drying and crumbling them up. You can also sometimes add herbal essential oils to the blend, but you have to make sure you aren't using an oil that's a skin irritant. Oregano, basil, thyme and nutmeg are all oils you're probably going to want to avoid, amongst others.

Here are a handful of herbal bath salt recipes to get you started.

Rosemary Bath Salts

This recipe calls for both dried rosemary and rosemary essential oil. Rosemary essential oil is a popular essential oil that smells like a stronger version of the herb used in cooking. It is thought to boost mental acuity, may relieve respiratory conditions and may even numb aches and pains. It can also be used to regulate sebum production and can be used to help alleviate oily skin.

Ingredients:

4 cups natural bath salt
15 drops of rosemary essential oil
1 tablespoon dried rosemary, crumbled

Directions:

1. Stir the rosemary essential oil into the salt until the essential oil has completely dispersed into the salts.
2. Add the dried rosemary and stir it in.
3. Spread the salts out and let them dry.
4. Store them in a nonreactive container in a cool, dry place.

Rosemary Mint Bath Salts

Add mint to the previous recipe and you get a potent bath salt blend that can be used to kill bacterial and fungal infections and is a natural remedy against respiratory conditions, congestion, colds and flus. Keep your time in the tub to a minimum when using this bath salt recipe.

Ingredients:

4 cups natural bath salt
10 drops of rosemary essential oil
5 drops peppermint essential oil
1 tablespoon dried rosemary, crumbled

Directions:

1. Combine the rosemary and the peppermint essential oil.
2. Stir the essential oil blend into the salt until the essential oil blend has completely dispersed into the salts.
3. Add the dried rosemary and stir it in.
4. Spread the salts out and let them dry.
5. Store them in a nonreactive container in a cool, dry place.

Focus Blend

This blend is a good choice when you need clarity of mind and are looking to focus on the tasks you need to accomplish. It's a great bath salt blend to use at the beginning of the day. You'll feel refreshed and ready to tackle anything life throws your way.

Ingredients:

4 cups natural bath salt
10 drops rosemary essential oil.
5 drops lemon essential oil.

Directions:

1. Stir the lemon essential oil and rosemary essential oil together.
2. Stir the oil blend into the salt until the essential oil has completely dispersed into the salts.
3. Spread the salts out and let them dry.
4. Store them in a nonreactive container in a cool, dry place.

Chapter 10: Citrus Salts

Citrus salts add the fragrance of citrus fruits to bath salts to create what I like to call "fruity salts." When it comes to using essential oils to create fruity salts, you're largely limited to citrus fruits, with maybe a small handful of other fruits being available occasionally.

This is where fragrance oils come into play, as there are synthetic oil blends available that can be used to make your bath salts smell like pretty much any fruit you can imagine. I'm not a big fan of fragrance oils, but will use them on occasion when an appropriate essential oil or oil blend isn't available.

Pink Grapefruit Bath Salts

I don't know what I like more about this bath salt recipe; the fact that it smells like pink grapefruit or the fact that it's naturally colored pink because Himalayan pink salts are used in the recipe.

Grapefruit essential oil is an uplifting oil that can lift your spirits when you're feeling down in the dumps. It has a fresh citrus fragrance, and it's a great oil when it comes to taking care of your skin. It's packed full of antioxidants, which helps prevent free radical damage to the skin. To top things off, it's good for your hair and will give it a lustrous, beautiful shine.

Ingredients:

4 cups Himalayan pink salt
15 drops grapefruit essential oil
1 tablespoon fresh grapefruit juice

Directions:

1. Combine the fresh grapefruit juice and the grapefruit essential oil.
2. Stir the grapefruit essential oil/juice mix into the salt until it's thoroughly mixed into the salt.
3. Spread the salts out and let them dry.
4. Store them in a nonreactive container in a cool, dry place.

Lemon Lime Bath Salts

This recipe combines fresh lime juice with lemon essential oil to create a refreshing fragrance that's rejuvenating and may even help tighten up the skin and remove or lessen minor wrinkles. I used to combine both lime and lemon essential oil, but have decided I like the way this recipe smells better.

Ingredients:

4 cups natural bath salt
10 drops of lemon essential oil
1 tablespoon fresh lime juice

Directions:

1. Combine the lime juice and lemon essential oil.
2. Stir the blend into the salt until the oil blend has completely dispersed into the salts.
3. Spread the salts out and let them dry.
4. Store them in a nonreactive container in a cool, dry place.

Lemon Seaweed Salts

Combining lemon essential oil with organic dried seaweed creates a luxurious bath that helps detoxify the skin and leaves you feeling great.

Ingredients:

4 cups natural bath salt
15 drops lemon essential oil
Dried organic seaweed.

Directions:

1. Stir the lemon essential oil into the salt until the essential oil has completely dispersed into the salts.
2. Crumble the dried seaweed. Add it to the bath salts and stir it in.
3. Spread the salts out and let them dry.
4. Store them in a nonreactive container in a cool, dry place.

Minty Lime Salts

Here's a great-smelling bath salt blend that will leave you feeling fresh and smelling like a mint mojito, minus the alcohol of course.

Ingredients:

4 cups natural bath salt
2 tablespoons lime juice
10 to 15 drops peppermint essential oil

Directions:

1. Stir the lime essential oil and lime juice into the salt until the essential oil has completely dispersed into the salts.
2. Spread the salts out and let them dry.
3. Store them in a nonreactive container in a cool, dry place.

Invigorating Citrus Bath Blend

Bergamot oil, which smells like oranges, is combined with grapefruit essential oil to create a refreshing bath salt blend that can be used in the bath in the morning when you've got a long day ahead and want to get it started right. It probably isn't the best blend to use in the evening when you're trying to wind down.

Ingredients:

4 cups natural bath salt
10 drops of Bergamot essential oil
5 drops of grapefruit essential oil

Directions:

1. Combine the Bergamot and the grapefruit essential oil.
2. Stir the essential oil blend into the salt until the essential oil blend has completely dispersed into the salts.
3. Spread the salts out and let them dry.
4. Store them in a nonreactive container in a cool, dry place.

Chapter 10: Juniper Sore Muscle Relief Bath Salts

If you've got sore muscles from a hard day's work or and you want some relief from the pain, juniper essential oil might be all it takes to soothe your aches and pains. It's also good for the skin and is a great-smelling essential oil that smells like juniper trees. I've seen juniper oil used as a relaxing and stress-relieving oil as well.

Ingredients:

4 cups natural bath salt
10 to 20 drops of juniper essential oil

Directions:

1. Stir the juniper essential oil into the salt until the essential oil has completely dispersed into the salts.
2. Spread the salts out and let them dry.
3. Store them in a nonreactive container in a cool, dry place.

Chapter 11: Vanilla Bath Salts

The first recipe in this chapter is a simple one. It only requires two ingredients and leaves your tub smelling like vanilla. I rarely make this recipe on its own, but I have been known to make it and add other essential oils to the mix.

<u>**Vanilla Bath Salts Recipe**</u>

Ingredients:

4 cups natural bath salt
2 tablespoons vanilla extract

Directions:

1. Stir the vanilla extract into the salt until it has completely dispersed into the salts.
2. Spread the salts out and let them dry.
3. Store them in a nonreactive container in a cool, dry place.

Vanilla Rose Bath Salts Recipe

This recipe is my go-to bath salt recipe when I'm looking for an awesome gift that people will love. I've seen recipes that call for vanilla fragrance oil, and you can use it if you want a strong artificial vanilla smell, but I prefer to use vanilla extract in this recipe.

As far as the rose oil goes, it's one of the more expensive essential oils, but you're only going to need a small amount for each batch of bath salts, and a little bit goes a long way. If you don't want to spend the money on rose essential oil, try one of the other floral oils instead. Lavender, geranium and jasmine oil will all work as well.

Ingredients:

4 cups natural bath salt
10 drops of rose essential oil
2 tablespoons dried rose petals, crumbled
1 tablespoon vanilla extract.

Directions:

1. Combine the vanilla and the rose essential oil.
2. Stir the essential oil blend into the salt until the essential oil blend has completely dispersed into the salts.
3. Add the dried rose petals and stir them in.
4. Spread the salts out and let them dry.
5. Store them in a nonreactive container in a cool, dry place.

Chapter 12: Cinnamon Oatmeal Bath Salts

This recipe doesn't call for any essential oils for fragrancing. You might be able to use cinnamon essential oil, but it's a fairly hot oil and not everyone can tolerate it, so I'd be cautious.

The cinnamon fragrance in this recipe comes from ground cinnamon, which has antibacterial and antifungal properties. The oatmeal turns the bath into a creamy, luxurious bath that will leave your skin feeling silky smooth.

If you want to make the bath water feel even better, try adding ½ a cup of powdered milk to this recipe as well. The lactic acid in the milk will help exfoliate your skin, and you'll be able to get rid of a lot of the dead skin cells you've got clinging to your body.

Ingredients:

4 cups natural bath salt
3 tablespoons ground cinnamon
1 cup oatmeal

Directions:

1. Grind the oatmeal until it's broken into fine particles.
2. Combine all of the ingredients and stir them together.

3. Store this recipe in a nonreactive container in a cool, dry place.

Chapter 13: Bubbling Bath Salts

The fragrance you use is up to you with this recipe. The glycerin soap base creates a nice bubble bath when you add the salts while you're filling the tub. As far as the fragrance goes, you can use any of the essential oils outlined thus far in the book.

Ingredients:

4 cups natural bath salt
½ cup liquid glycerin soap base
2 tablespoons sweet almond oil
10 to 20 drops of your favorite essential oils or oil blend

Directions:

1. Combine the glycerin soap base, almond oil and any essential oils you plan on adding.
2. Add the mixture to the salts and stir until they're coated.
3. Spread the salts out and let them dry.
4. Store them in an airtight container in a cool, dry place.

Chapter 14: Detoxification Bath Salts

This recipe can be used to help pull toxins out of the body and to cleanse the skin. If you're experiencing skin issues like minor rashes and infections, this bath might be able to help alleviate those conditions. One thing's for sure. This bath is extremely relaxing, so it's probably a bad idea to use the detox salts in the morning when you've got a long day ahead. They're more appropriate for use in the evening when you're trying to wind down.

Try adding half a cup of apple cider vinegar to the bath for an extra detox boost. Don't worry about the smell…You can cover it with essential oils. It goes away quickly and won't leave you smelling like vinegar.

The essential oils used are up to you. The following oils are thought to help with detoxification:

- **Grapefruit.**
- **Lavender.**
- **Lemon.**
- **Patchouli.**
- **Peppermint.**
- **Rosemary.**

Detox Bath Salts

Ingredients:

4 cups Himalayan pink salt
1 cup baking soda
½ cup Epsom salt
15 to 20 drops of your favorite essential oils or oil blend

Directions:

1. Combine the Himalayan pink salt, baking soda and Epsom salt in a bowl.
2. Add the essential oil to the salts and stir until they're coated.
3. Spread the salts out and let them dry.
4. Store them in an airtight container in a cool, dry place.

Bentonite Clay Bath

This recipe adds bentonite clay to the mix. This natural clay pulls toxins and heavy metals out of the body and will leave you feeling fresh and clean. You only need to use these bath salts once a month to reap the benefits of the clay.

Ingredients:

4 cups natural bath salt
1 cup bentonite clay
10 to 20 drops of your favorite essential oils or oil blend

Directions:

1. Combine the bath salts and the bentonite clay.
2. Add the essential oils to the salt and clay mixture and stir until combined.
3. Spread the salts out and let them dry.
4. Store them in an airtight container in a cool, dry place.

Chapter 15: Sleepy Time Salt Blend

Do you have trouble going to sleep at night?

Bath salts alone might be enough to help you wind down. The essential oils used in this bath salt blend have an almost-narcotic effect and should help you drift off to sleep shortly after taking a bath with these bath salts.

This should go without saying, but this isn't a blend you're going to want to use at the start of a long day. Save this one for those nights where you're wound up and are having trouble drifting off to sleep.

Sleepy Time Salt Blend Recipe

Ingredients:

4 cups natural bath salt
10 drops lavender essential oil
5 drops cedarwood essential oil
5 drops patchouli essential oil
5 drops Roman chamomile essential oil

Directions:

1. Combine the essential oils.
2. Add the mixture to the salts and stir until they're coated.
3. Spread the salts out and let them dry.
4. Store them in an airtight container in a cool, dry place.

Lavender Sleepy Time Blend

This blend is probably mild enough to where it can be used to help older children wind down, but make sure you check with your physician prior to using it, and be sure to only use a small amount of the salts.

Ingredients:

4 cups natural bath salt
2 tablespoons sweet almond oil
10 drops lavender essential oil

Directions:

1. Combine the essential oil and sweet almond oil.
2. Add the mixture to the salts and stir until they're coated.
3. Spread the salts out and let them dry.
4. Store them in an airtight container in a cool, dry place.

Using Bath Salts

Bath salts are easy to use. All you have to do is fill the tub up partway with warm water and then toss a cup or two of the bath salts into the running water. The running water will help disperse the bath salts into the tub and they'll be dissolved almost instantly.

Once the salts have dissolved into the tub water, climb in and soak for a while. The length of time you should soak depends on how strong the essential oil blend you used is and how much bath salts were added to the tub. Most people soak 15 to 30 minutes when they've added bath salts to the tub.

You can also use bath salts for exfoliation of dead skin. Grab a handful of bath salts and add a little water to them. Rub the mixture into the area you want to exfoliate and it should eliminate dead skin cells, leaving your skin feeling soft and supple.

Printed in Great Britain
by Amazon

23930093R00036